LAUGH
OUT LOUD

LAUGH
OUT LOUD

YOUR PERSONAL PRESCRIPTION FOR
THE BEST MEDICINE ON EARTH

JACK DALY

LAUGH OUT LOUD

Your Personal Prescription for the Best Medicine on Earth

For more information, email: jack@laughoutloud.info

Copyright Number: TXu 2-400-207

Paperback ISBN: 979-8-9894872-0-2

eBook ISBN: 979-8-9894872-1-9

Audiobook ISBN: 979-8-9894872-2-6

Library of Congress Control Number: 2023921935

Get Your Free Gift!

To get the best experience with this book, I've found readers who download and use the *LAUGH OUT LOUD* Audiobook can implement faster and take the next steps needed to put a smile on your face, a ray of sunshine in your heart, and some happiness in your life.

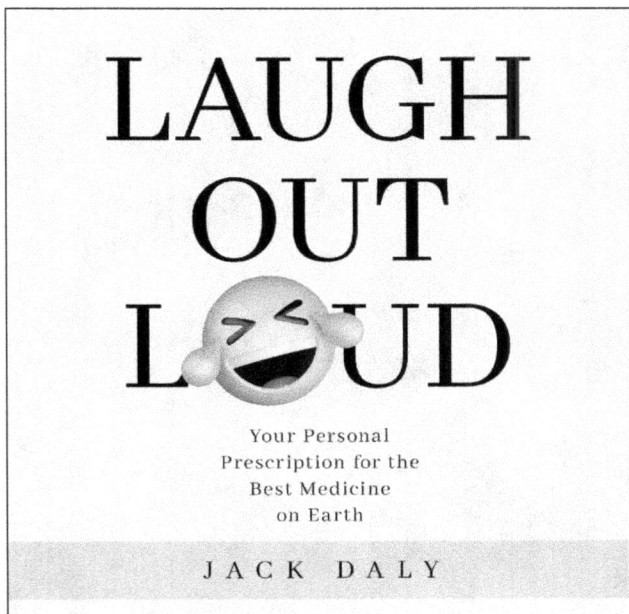

Pre-order your FREE copy by visiting:

www.laughoutloudbook.com

Dedication

To my loving wife, Andrea, for whom,
without her belief in me, encouragement, love,
and sugar-free support, this book would not exist.

Foreword

In our complex world, brimming with challenges, laughter's healing potential is often overlooked, especially in times of adversity. Jack Daly's *"Laugh Out Loud"* introduces a refreshing, practical five-step approach, seamlessly integrating laughter into personal growth, resilience, and healing.

Jack's method, both simple and profound, fosters a mindset where laughter naturally counterbalances life's challenges, underscoring its vital role in personal development. This book transcends mere humor; it's a roadmap to cultivating resilience through laughter as a daily, intentional practice.

Endorsing *"Laugh Out Loud,"* I invite you to explore and harness laughter's transformative power. Jack's insights provide us with a new perspective to enrich our life journey, advocating laughter not just as a source of transient joy, but as a steadfast ally in overcoming life's hurdles. It's an invitation to find peace and solidarity, turning life's challenges into opportunities for growth and connection.

Mirthfully yours,
Sebastian Gendry
Laughter Online University

Table of Contents

Blue <u>underlined</u> text in the book equates to a URL address in the Resources section on page 65.

INTRODUCTION

"Trouble knocked at the door, but,
hearing laughter hurried away."
- Benjamin Franklin

Humanity is in a state of crisis and despair on a global scale. All of humanity is under threat, unlike we've ever known. Despots are everywhere we turn, sowing and spewing their evil. Our children are now their prey, targeted as young as five and six years old in the classroom. Parents are being told they have no right to make decisions for their own children and that it is the state's right and responsibility. Gender dysphoria is being exploited for monetary gain and fame. Communication is being weaponized on every medium available to society. Brainwashing is occurring around the globe in every walk of life. Despair and hopelessness abound given that the world is still reeling from one of the most tragic events, the COVID-19 Pandemic; its impact devastating in numerous ways, fuelled with deception and deceit. Add to this the ever-corrupt political strife stretching to the four corners of the globe. The wars in Israel and Ukraine and the threat of war in the Pacific could potentially become another world war with weapons of mass destruction in the hands of

1

certifiable madmen and incompetents. Personal and national security is in its most insecure state ever in history. Daily headlines focus on all things negative, few and far between which accentuate the positive. Say nothing of the day-to-day stressors in life that we face.

My apologies for the reality check.

In this book, I provide a tool, a guide, for use in your daily life. At the very least, it offers a glimmer of hope, a distraction, a respite. It is something to grasp with both hands and cherish to enhance your well-being and ease your mind during these critically troubling times. We each face numerous conditions daily that tax our souls and test our existence. At times, these can be overwhelming; all we seek is a way out. *Laugh Out Loud* may not be a way out, but it is a way to cope daily if practiced.

Laughter is like sunshine for the soul; it cleanses the mind and invigorates the body inside and out. When a person enjoys a good chuckle, beneficial reactions occur within the body, boosting numerous vital processes. Laughing acts as a form of low-impact exercise, burning calories, regulating blood pressure, reducing pain, increasing oxygen intake (that's a good one!), and boosting the immune system. Not too shabby, huh? So, the next time you tell a coworker a joke, remember that you're probably doing them a greater favor than any doctor or pharmacist could. Practice these five steps and live happier. Each day, complete these steps of L.A.U.G.H., I promise you won't regret it.

I will unequivocally state here in writing for all the world to see that having the ability to laugh helped keep my head above water during my most profound, darkest moments of despair when I thought I would be swallowed up whole or drown in my tears. Whether laughing humoristically or sarcastically didn't matter. It served as my lifeline. Regardless of the situation you may be experiencing at any given moment in time, there is one thing that every man, woman, and child on earth experiences, even if just for a fleeting moment: the sense of happiness when laughing or hearing someone else laugh. It's magical in how it can transform one from feeling desperate to feeling hopeful in a matter of seconds.

With this guide, I aim to arm you with my weapon of choice for facing life's daunting challenges, whether significant or minor, real or perceived. Although it may not initially be evident to some, this practice can be empowering and perhaps even lead to an awakening. In my own life, I learned at an early age that life was far more enjoyable and happier than unhappy, despite the many sad times I experienced. Some were of my own making, while others were entirely beyond my control. Regardless, I strived to find a thread of humor in even the unpleasant scenarios, not to make light of them, but not to permit them to be dark or overwhelming, thus, how *Laugh Out Loud* came to be for you.

Did I succeed in every case? No. I forced myself to find a reason or a higher purpose in situations where no thread of humor was found. Did I manage to find an excuse or a higher purpose in each of those situations? Again, no. Some had to be accepted for what they were, and I had to move forward, trying not to look back—which can be incredibly hard sometimes. I find it therapeutic to reflect on the happy moments and situations, especially those that still make me laugh, even if it's just for a few seconds. It's therapy for the heart, mind, and soul that you won't find on any drugstore shelf. In life, there is but one choice that impacts our lives with a ripple effect like a stone thrown into a pond: the choice of happiness.

I promise that following the five steps outlined in this guide will bring a smile to your face, a ray of sunshine to your heart, and, at the very least, a moment (if not several) of happiness to your life. I have written this guide to share a daily ritual that has been my secret weapon. In facing my challenges, I have repeatedly found laughter to be an unstoppable force with no counter device or method to defeat it. With absolute confidence, I can say there never will be one. However, the ability to laugh will become your own personal countermeasure.

- Waiting for What?! -

Don't deny yourself and others a moment of laughter and happiness. Being happy is a choice every one of us has at our disposal. Happiness can be fleeting; however, laughter can be infectious. Declared life's best medicine, get your prescription now! Why wait?! I'm not an M.D., but I will write you this prescription regardless! Now, let's read *Laugh Out Loud! It's your very own personal prescription for the best medicine on earth!*

*I*T'S A PROCESS (but of course it is)

"The most wasted of all days is one without laughter."
- E. E. Cummings

- The Sweetest Sound You'll Ever Hear -

A child's laughter ranks among the earth's most enchanting sounds. I vividly recall the day I first heard my infant daughter's genuine belly laugh. She was a mere three-month-old, resting on my thighs as I lounged on the sofa, my feet propped up on the coffee table. As I gazed into Jessie's baby-blue eyes—wide with wonder at the world, including the sight of me chatting and playing with her plump arms and legs—someone on the TV blurted, "Reach for the sky." Intrigued, I mimicked the barrel of a pistol with my index finger, aimed it at Jessie, and echoed the line: "Reach for the sky," anticipating no particular response. Her reaction was unexpected: a rich, deep belly giggle that caught me off guard and sparked my unrestrained laughter, tears streaming down my face. Emboldened, I tried again. "Reach for the sky," I repeated, and Jessie's laughter grew even more boisterous. I chuckled until I was sore while she resumed her curious exploration with those inquisitive baby blues. In that moment, I savored the sweetest sound I'd ever heard: my child's laughter—a symphony to my ears.

It's a memory I revisit for a spiritual lift, which never fails to elevate me.

As time has unfolded and my family has grown with the additions of Tim and Erin, the melodious laughter of my children has been a source of constant joy for my ears, heart, mind, and soul.

The Navajo honor a baby's first chuckle with the "First Laugh Ceremony" (A'wee Chi'deedloh), which celebrates the belief that with their initial laughter, children become beings ready to embrace life and love, transitioning from the spiritual world into humanity.

Throughout my life, I have reveled in the laughter of children far and wide. A particularly cherished memory is a Pepsi commercial from Christmases past, likely unscripted, capturing the pure joy of spontaneity. The commercial featured a young boy, perhaps four or five years old, engulfed in a litter of ebullient yellow Labrador retriever puppies. As they jumped, clambered, and licked him, his squeals of delight were infectious. I, too, laughed heartily, tears accompanying each guffaw. Every viewing elicited the same heartfelt response, undoubtedly shared by countless others. I often wish I could have been behind the camera, witnessing the length of that boy's glee. I imagine it left everyone on set—and perhaps many viewers—revisiting that harmonious laughter in their hearts for years to come.

-You Need to be Infected -

The best infection you could ever ask for? What?! Wait a minute, have you lost your mind? Do you want another infection with COVID going around?! YES, you do! You NEED it —today and every day for the rest of your life. It might be the very thing that keeps you alive. I am not jesting with this statement. As I mentioned in the introduction, being able to laugh served as my lifeline in the most trying times. I use the word 'infectious' as a descriptor for laughter because it is an act one can choose to engage in or not. However, sometimes you have no choice; no matter how valiant your effort to resist or suppress it, you're going to lose. It's just like Stilwell, the bratty kid in "A League of Their Own[1]," taunted, "you're gonna lose," and there are no two ways about it.

Just hearing someone else laughing their ass off (what a great weight loss idea) can make the sourest of a human being fall apart at the seams laughing. I remember one evening in the Crew Team dorm at Florida Institute of Technology (FIT) when Jim V. and I watched a movie, and the Freshman Team coach, Steve W., talked on the payphone in our living room. I had no idea who Steve (a born funny guy) was talking to, but he started laughing uncontrollably at whatever (we never learned). His laughter made us laugh so hard we cried, tears rolling down our cheeks with our sides splitting. It was the most joyous torture we would ever know at the time...just sitting here chronicling it has me cracking up. I laughed myself to sleep that night. Try that one on for a change instead of sex—well, maybe only if you are single and alone, or you could end up being so. I don't recommend it during or immediately following lovemaking unless you've decided you like financially supporting some divorce lawyer.

On occasion (okay, on *many*), my laughter has come at the expense of another, even my wife. It just so happens I love Halloween, and what better time for a prankster at heart like me? See, my wife, Andrea, suffers from a case of arachnophobia and hates spiders with a passion, amongst other crawling and scampering little creatures. Oh, what a cornucopia of scary opportunities for me on this mysterious night every 31st of October! It's amazing the screams a bag full of rubber arachnids and other creepy crawlers can elicit

7

in the bedroom. Beware, you will (not might) end up like me, sleeping on the couch in the basement with the real creepy crawlers for the price of your amusement.

Laughter is resounding, so why not do it? Go ahead—I triple-dog dare ya—go Laugh Out Loud!

Do you want to be happy, even just a little each day? Then, choose to be. It's up to you and you alone.

How you choose to implement and practice the following five steps of the Laugh Out Loud practice is also entirely up to you:

Step-1: *L*augh

Step-2: *A*ct

Step-3: *U*nplug

Step-4: *G*row

Step-5: *Humor (me/us)*

All five steps are designed to be completed in one hour, for an average of 12 minutes (60 minutes divided by five steps) each. However, you can choose how much time you want to dedicate to each step. Set a timer to stay on track. OK, who has a spare hour in their day, you ask—then I ask you if *one hour* out of your day is worth spending on yourself, to improve your life. Even if you feel your life is perfect or needs no improvement, a little pick-me-up never hurts. It's your choice. Throughout this process, I'm your coach, not your judge, jury, or executioner.

Pressed for time today, as we all are at times, which seems all too often to be the case these days, then you can knock out the five steps of *L*augh-*A*ct-*U*nplug-*G*row-*Humor (me/us)* (*L.A.U.G.H*) in five minutes spending one minute on each.

The benefits of even one minute per step will be beneficial, if for no other reason than you step back from the toils of the day to take five minutes to come up for air, relax, and enjoy a good chuckle, guffaw, or giggle and de-stress. Take this mini vacation once daily or as many times as you need for your sanity and well-being. Laughter has been proven to have psychological and physical positive effects on humans. In a 1988 study commissioned by Norman Cousins, editor of the Saturday Review, researchers confirmed that laughter reduces cortisol, an immunosuppressant hormone, in the blood. Their findings were published in the American Journal of Medical Sciences[2]. They stated, "The study has shown objective, measurable, and significant neuroendocrine and stress hormone changes with mirthful laughter," they wrote, noting that laughter "can reverse or attenuate" hormonal changes brought on by stress. Several years later, they reported that laughter increases natural-killer cell production, which helps the body fight allergies, cancer, diabetes, and heart disease.

The beauty of this daily ritual, and I highly recommend you make it a daily practice, is to reap its maximum benefits that it's flexible. How much time you dedicate to practice is your choice—seeing a pattern here? What's my recommendation? If you don't have 60 minutes to spare, give it half the time; 30 minutes is what I recommend. Most of us get at least 30 minutes for a lunch break. Take advantage of the time you have to yourself. You can do all but one of the steps and eat your lunch at the same time, even the *Act* step, which, if exercising, you can eat a sandwich while walking and taking in a beautiful day, which allows you to *Unplug* at the same time.

STEP-1

LAUGH - To Your Heart's Content

"As soap is to the body, so laughter is to the soul."
- Jewish Proverb

CAUTION/DISCLAIMER: *Do not* do Step-1 Laugh while eating. You could be a new statistic, the evening news headline reading, they died laughing (and choked to death) eating a ham sandwich (with mustard and pickles), and I go to jail for killing you with laughter!

But seriously, folks, don't try to chew and laugh at the same time. To begin with, it's not pretty, and no one else around you desires to wear your lunch when you shower them with your egg and quinoa salad (with jalapenos).

Laughing is contagious, the best pandemic the world could ever hope for. Laugh as often and hardily as you want, and you'll infect others with the best bug in the world.

Remember from the previous chapter the mental and physical benefits of laughing and the physiological changes that result within you? Of note is the reversal of the harmful chemical effects of stress. A *Mayo Clinic Staff n.d.* report[3] states, "Negative thoughts manifest into chemical reactions that can affect your body by bringing more stress into your system and decreasing your immunity. By contrast, positive thoughts can release neuropeptides that help fight stress and potentially more serious illnesses." Laughing is an excellent hefty dose of neuropeptides for the mind, heart, body, and soul. Without a doubt, it is the world's best medicine!

The social benefits of laughing are invaluable when you share your laughter with others. With all the divisiveness in the world today, laughing serves as an international language without saying a single word. It conveys the most potent message no world leader can deny, even the despot.

Find something funny or silly to laugh out loud about— anything that cracks you up!

Some ideas for a good laugh:

- Personal Photo or Memory -

Sometimes personal photos or home movies are the best, especially if they involve a family member. Not only are they humorous, but they are endearing memories, making them even more special. Have you ever done something so embarrassing you were mortified if anyone witnessed or heard your gaff and you wanted to disappear into thin air, yet hours later, you laughed about it? Of course, you have; we all have. It made the embarrassment a little easier to handle. You accepted your mistake or misstep and moved on, acknowledging that you are human and that no one is perfect, despite what some people may think of themselves. One of my own is coming up.

- JibJab Video -

You can make a JibJab video with you in it. Being able to laugh at yourself is the highest form of self-confidence.

- YouTube Videos -

The all-time classics of funny people like Johnny Carson with Robin Williams[4], Andy Kaufman, Sam Kennison, Jonathan Winters, Don Rickles, or Foster Brooks, and the Dean Martin Roasts (not PC by today's cockeyed standards). How about reruns of *Two and a Half Men* for a good laugh? YouTube videos of these comics were some of the funniest things I have ever seen and heard in my life. Two of my all-time favorites were Robin Williams, one of the funniest men ever to live, (rest in peace, good sir) and Tim Conway. Hundreds, maybe even thousands of YouTube videos will split your sides with laughter. Another one of my favorites of all time is little Rose in her car seat trying to unbuckle the straps holding her in. Her father sees what she is doing, and he very politely asks if there is anything he can do to assist (not that he's going to unbuckle her while driving down the road). Her reply is entirely unexpected for a child who, at most, is maybe three years old.

"Worry about yourself—worry about yourself," declares Rose, trying to escape the binds of her car seat.

"Can I help?" asks her father (in the driver's seat).

"You want me to help," Dad inquires again.

"No…no thank you," says Rose.

"What do you want me to do?" he asks.

"Worry about yourself, worry about yourself," Rose retorts.

13

"Are you sure? asks her father.

"No, you drive the car—take care of yourself," she declares… her dad starts to crack up but tries to hold it in—not with much luck, mind you.

"Are you sure?" he inquires again.

Indignantly, Rose replies, "You drive the car—take care of yourself!" Her father loses it at this point and is cracking up, desperate not to encourage her behavior by laughing too loudly.

It's so innocent it makes it all the funnier, and I never tire of watching it.

There are many other professional comedians like George Lopez, Larry the Cable Guy, Jeff Foxworthy, Chris Rock, Tina Fey, Larry David, Amy Poehler, Dave Chappelle, and Rodney Dangerfield, to name a few. Then there are the everyday people, non-professional comedians who do or say things—sometimes unintentional—that are just so darn side-splitting funny you can't help but laugh, even at some of the dumb things a human being can say or do.

- **Old Skit** "Who's on First?" – The old classic skit by Bud Abbott and Lou Costello is impossible not to laugh at, regardless of how many times you have heard it.

- **Facebook Group** "Jokes of the Day" – Someone posts a hilarious joke (or several) on this FB page every day. Some ask you to post your response, such as using the word "testicles" in the title of one of your favorite movies. My reply to that one, *"A Few Good Testicles,"* with Tom Cruise and Jack Nicholson.

- Cartoons -

One of my all-time favorites is "The Far Side" – cartoons. They mix humor, sarcasm, and a bit of reality, which results in them being all the funnier. People send some of the most humorous cartoons via email, sometimes containing everything from animals to politics. Some are just plain dumb (which can be funny), and others can have you rolling on the floor laughing like an idiot.

The above are just a few ideas on how to have yourself a good laugh, and there are many, many more. What can you think of to bust a gut laughing? What's your favorite? Use it as your go-to for a good chuckle to brighten up your day!

Personally, I love making others laugh as much as I love laughing myself—especially since I don't think I'm all that funny, but my wife thinks I am, and that's all that counts, right guys? A happy wife equals a happy life!

Have you ever told someone that you 'died laughing' after hearing a joke or seeing something so funny that you couldn't control yourself, perhaps even confessing that you peed your pants? I know I have—as a kid, the yellow snow was proof enough, not to mention the wet spot on the front of my pants, as wide as the Grand Canyon. OK, that's the only confession you'll get out of me in this book! Come on! We've all done something that at that moment was the most embarrassing thing we've ever done...but later in life...we laughed our asses off over it, at least to ourselves in private or with a close confidant.

- Comedy Audio Tracks -

Comedy routines of every genre and comedian from the 21st century are archived in audio recording format of one type or another, whether on vinyl albums (aka LPs), 8-track or cassette tapes, or today via music apps for iTunes and Apple Music for iPhones and iPads or via Amazon Music for Android devices, to mention a few. Download your favorites to your device, and you can have the experience as often as you desire. Even better, you can share the laughter with whomever you choose. Be careful with the sharing; it could come back to bite you—it did me.

The first comedy album/LP (long-playing format) I ever listened to was in high school while a sophomore at West Catholic for Boys in Philadelphia, Pennsylvania. In the West Philadelphia area where I lived, it was one of the larger Catholic high schools in the region. The key here is it was a Catholic school. Yep, I'm an Irish Catholic (Kat-lick). The album in question was George Carlin's *Class Clown,* perfect for a kid in high school to listen to, right? What could be bad about it? Oh, you have no idea…I'll explain. There were (still are) numerous questionable tracks in *Class Clown* with which the Catholic Church would have issues.

I had to confess to listening to them on Saturday afternoon before my soul would be cleansed appropriately by a priest under the sacrament of confession. The "Father" would then issue penance for committing the many sins I had just confessed to in the triple phone booth with the privacy screens before accepting Christ's body and blood into my gullet via the sacrament of Holy Communion on Sunday morning during Mass. Oh, this was the least of the penances I would have to bear. Here are just a couple of the sinful tracks I listened to from the famous George Carlin on that album: "I Used to Be Irish Catholic," "The Confessional," "Special Dispensation - Heaven, Hell, Purgatory and Limbo," "Heavy Mysteries," and the "Seven Words You Can Never Say on Television." It was excellent and the worst of them all—some of the funniest stuff I've ever heard.

16

So, by far the most sinful of all was the "Seven Words…" but the one I would pay hell for was "The Confessional." You see, at the time, I was dating my first real girlfriend, Ellen, who lived down the street from me in a five-story apartment building. Her father, Ed, was a friend of my father and they had known each other for years. Much like me, Ellen also lived with and was being raised by her grandmother, and naturally, both grandmothers knew each other as well. It gets worse. It was through Ellen's father that we met. See, I was cursed with being the boy every grandmother in the neighborhood wanted their granddaughters to date. Why? Because I was considered the nice, squeaky-clean boy in the neighborhood. Yeah, right. Squeaky clean? Ha! Don't make me laugh! Ellen had a younger brother, Vincent, who was a couple of years younger than me. My first sin was lending the album to Vinny, as friends and family called him. Despite having listened to the album in its entirety days before, I had data-dumped that there was part of a track regarding a girl named Ellen. Vinny, in his evil boyhood little-brother ways, chose to play that track, "The Confessional," during the Quinn family dinner with all present at the table—himself, Ellen, dad, and last but not least, grandmom. The track was benign until Mr. Carlin explained it was a sin to "wanna." If you woke up one morning and decided to rob the bank, he said to save your carfare—you just committed the sin because you "wanna."

Then, with Ellen's family listening intently, George stated the following:

"It's a sin to wanna feel up, Ellen,

it's a sin to plan to feel up, Ellen,

it's a sin to figure out a place to feel up, Ellen,

it's a sin to take Ellen to the place to feel her up,

17

it's a sin to try to feel her up,

and it's a sin to feel her up. It's six sins in one feel, man!"

I arrived shortly after the dinner dishes had been washed and put away, unaware of the ambush awaiting me that evening. As usual, I knocked on the door, anxious to see one of the hottest girls I'd ever laid eyes on at the ripe age of 15. The door opened, and BAM! There stood her grandmother, glaring at me with the worst stink-eye I had ever received, her face contorted with utter contempt as she uttered, "Oh, it's you."

"Good evening, Mrs. Q.," I responded, bewildered.

In the hallway, Vinny was grinning, with a bird's-eye view of the front door and the living room. "Jack, come in here, please," bellowed Ellen's father from the living room. *What the hell is going on?* raced through my mind as I turned the corner to enter the living room. There, Mr. Q., burly and imposing, sat in the wing-backed chair next to the window— my only escape route, four stories above the ground. To my left, Ellen sat on the sofa, her head down, staring at the carpet. *What the hell is going on?* I thought again. *What did I do?* Then, the interrogation commenced.

Mr. Q stared me right between the eyes and fired a full salvo like the battleship USS New Jersey.

"So Jack...why do you want to feel up my daughter Ellen?" he demanded.

"Huh—what—I don't want to feel her up (yes you do, dumb-ass declared my evil twin inside me)—why would you think that?" I asked, noticing her grandmother standing behind me, scowling as I looked to see if she was wielding a weapon, such as her thirteen-inch cast-iron skillet. With my knees weakening and my mouth dry as the Sahara Desert, I

18

stood on trial before my judge, jury, and executioner. Vinny was still standing in the same spot, his face beet red from suppressing his laughter. He was clearly getting a kick out of my torture. Then Mr. Q. pronounced my life sentence. I was sure I would be banished for life. Worse still, I anticipated a phone call from one irate grandmother to another—mine—who would be waiting for me to walk through the door. BAM! Ambush number two!

"Jack, that's some of the funniest stuff I've ever heard," declared Ellen's father, "You can relax now. You're not in any trouble. Vincent played that part for us during dinner."

Why, you little SOB, I thought as Mr. Q., Vincent, and Ellen laughed at my expense. Her grandmother, however, hadn't so much as grinned. Her scowl was ice cold, and I could feel the arctic chill in the air. I turned to look at Vinny with my icy scowl and said, "Thanks, pal." They had their laugh at my expense. For the rest of the evening, I didn't so much as even hold Ellen's hand in fear her grandmother would chop it off right there on the coffee table and send me home banished for life. Each time I remember that evening or hear that segment of *Class Clown,* I chuckle. It took me weeks to work up the nerve to even attempt to kiss Ellen. I finally did have my first kiss, out on the fire escape one Friday night, only to be caught by, of all people, her grandmother, who banished me from the apartment that night for weeks. It was worth the penalty I paid.

As you read this scenario, I'm sure you have experienced one growing up, which will come back to you. I hope you get a good laugh out of it, too.

Now, let's really get the blood flowing and shake your booty!

STEP-2

ACT - Get Your Blood Flowing from Physical Activity

"Your body cannot heal without play. Your mind cannot heal without laughter. Your soul cannot heal without joy."
- Catherine Rippenger Fenwick

In Step-1, the idea is to find something to laugh at or about—whatever gets you to crack up.

CAUTION/DISCLAIMER: As with any exercise, you must be aware of your limitations, especially if you have any underlying health conditions that would make exercising potentially harmful to your overall well-being. If in doubt, consult your physician for guidance. Even the laughing exercises described below could be something to get your doctor's advice about. Also, depending upon where you are, you may have to consider your safety if venturing beyond your home's or other dwelling's security.

The goal is to move your body and exercise your muscles and lungs. It gets the blood flowing as your heart rate increases and forces you to take in more oxygen than you would be doing for most normal activities. The benefits to your body, mind, and soul are invaluable. Exercising provides gratification and a sense of accomplishment, achievement, and success that carry over into your daily life. Exercise helps promote a healthy lifestyle, too. For those of us who struggle to keep our weight in check, exercising regularly aids us in this challenge.

You can exercise indoors or outdoors, with the latter being the better choice as it allows you to breathe fresh air, soak in the sunshine, which equates to vitamin D (and it's free), and enjoy the wide-open blue sky above, reminding you that there are no boundaries. Take a walk outside for all the obvious reasons mentioned. Additionally, it allows you to use your eyes and ears, helping refresh your mind.

There are hundreds of different ways to exercise. Choose your favorite activity that can be completed in 12 minutes or less. You can always adjust the timing of each step to fit your preferences, desires, and any time constraints. The crucial part is performing each step daily, even if you need to space them throughout the day. Consistency is most important during the five steps each day. Don't worry if you miss a day or take a day off. Even the Good Lord rested on the seventh day, so you can, too.

When's the best time to exercise? The answer to that question is multi-faceted for the individual, depending on their schedules, responsibilities, and preferences. I try to exercise in the morning on the back end of doing my "S.A.V.E.R.S." from The Miracle Morning[5] book by Hal Elrod, and before I sit down at the keyboard to write. Exercising in the morning before I write makes my mind work more efficiently, as it increases my blood flow. Additionally, getting it done early means I don't have the nagging feeling and associated guilt throughout the day about still needing to complete it.

- Laughter Online University -

Did you know that there are laughing exercises you can do anywhere you want? There is a laughter university that teaches one how to exercise through laughing. It's called Laughter Online University (LOU)[6] founded by Sebastian Gendry, a French-born American citizen who spent 20 years as a "corporate Jedi" to the point of two stress-induced burnouts in a brief period before realizing he was on the wrong path in life. Through his quest to find a better way of life, he traversed the globe. He attended training to become a "Laughter Yoga" instructor. The move changed his life for the better, not only for himself but for all he taught in 18 countries and those he teaches today—I just so happen to be one of his current students.

One of the highly valuable resources on the website is Sebastian's book, 505 Best of Laughter Exercises[7], covering everything from laughter affirmations to laughter yoga. The overall benefits of exercise are too numerous to mention here and have been documented by far more knowledgeable individuals in hundreds, if not thousands, of other books. However, it's undeniable that exercise is beneficial. Therefore, try to do it at least three times a week, if not more. Although it may be difficult initially, stick with it. The benefits are well worth your time and effort. If physically taxing exercises aren't your thing, consider trying laughing exercises. Why not have a chuckle while you exercise?

As a high school athlete, particularly in crew (also known as rowing or sculling), I usually exercised in the afternoons after school, except during spring break when we had twice-a-day practices. In the summer and following graduation, my practice schedule shifted to early mornings, typically being on the water by 5:30 a.m., and we returned to twice-a-day sessions as we prepared for the 1976 Junior World Rowing Championships in Villach, Austria. During my college years, most of my practice schedule was also in the early mornings. Thus, out of necessity, my body adapted to being a morning person. I remain one to this day, although I make sure to listen to my body and allow myself to sleep past 7:00 a.m. for one or two mornings if needed. Rowing was life-changing. It taught me discipline that carried over into other positive aspects of my life, which I still adhere to.

- Not a Fan of Exercise? -

If, for whatever reason, you are not an exerciser, physical exercise is not the only thing you can do to accomplish this step. There are numerous ways to *Act*. For instance, volunteer to help someone less fortunate or limited in mobility. It can be as simple as helping an older adult load their groceries in their car or aid them in crossing the street, but be careful not to take a handbag filled with quarters to the head. Offer to clean someone's house who may be less than capable. Prepare a meal for the single-parent family working full-time and juggling the care and feeding of multiple children. Why not offer to assist the neighbor caring for an ill loved one whose garden is overgrown or whose house needs light repairs? What about your housework or repairs that will get you moving and exercise your muscles.

One of the most rewarding workouts I've ever experienced in my lifetime wasn't in a gym or a racing shell—it was doing a good deed. One December day in 2022, along with my wife, Andrea, we spent the afternoon loading Santa bags full of toys into cars of families challenged financially. We undertook this task in support of the U.S. Marine Corps-sponsored "Toys for Tots" program. Good people from the area donated toys to children so they would have a joyous morning on Christmas day with presents under the tree. Volunteers from across the community collected, transported, sorted, and bagged the toys for the children through a process that rivals any assembly line. Many of the vehicles that drove up to the delivery point had children inside who appeared somewhat confused about the big red bags being loaded into the trunk of their mother's or father's car. I knew their confusion would vanish in a split second when they saw the brightly wrapped and tied packages under the boughs of a beautifully decorated tree. I imagined the looks on their faces on Christmas morning, at the very least, smiles stretching from ear to ear. It filled my heart with joy. What a great way to burn off some calories!

- Take a Hike -

Go for a walk. It is far less strenuous than training for a marathon but still has significant health benefits. Walking not only exercises the muscles but also the mind. Breathing the fresh air alone benefits the mind, body, and soul. While walking, let your mind conjure up other ways to enhance your health within your limits, or decide to break some of your self-imposed barriers, maybe even laugh at them along the way.

What's your favorite way to get your blood flowing? I'll bet many of you answer with a three-letter word!

Now get off your butt and *move!*

STEP-3

*U*NPLUG - Put That Darn Thing Down

"I see skies of blue and clouds of white, the bright blessed days…and I think to myself, what a wonderful world."
- Louis Armstrong

In Step 2 - *A*ct, the basic idea was to get you physically moving and your blood flowing for all the helpful benefits it brings you.

- Breaking News -

Casket makers report a marked increase in orders from undertakers for caskets with a large, raised bubble in the lid for those who died with their head down looking at a cell phone and for men who overdosed on Viagra. Obviously, the cause of death dictates the location of the bubble.

Social interaction through human face-to-face encounters are starting to go the way of the Model-T Ford—that's no joke. I use the extreme here, because it is proven that with the advent of technology, social interaction has taken a back seat to the evolution or invention of the next-generation device. Add the social distancing forced upon the world by the COVID-19 pandemic. We now have children who can't make the grade in school because they were isolated from other children—critical in their formative years.

Communicating with auditory tools (ears and mouth) we are all born with is being replaced by thumbs. Instead of dialing the phone to speak to a friend or family member, texting is the most chosen communication path. Texting is used in place of speech to say hello, announce an achievement, convey anger, or whatever would have typically been spoken ten years ago. It's even being used for sexual gratification via "sexting." How far is this going to go?

The dangers of texting and driving are staggering! The United States National Highway Traffic Safety Administration[8], reports that cell phone use while driving led to 377 fatal crashes and 28,994 people were injured in 2021.

Turn off your devices: iPhones, iPads, iWatches, Androids, cell phones, TVs, radios, and so on.

- Meditate -

Find a meditation you can do independently without using any electronic device, recite a poem or prayer, or even your favorite nursery rhyme you loved as a child. I've personally found meditation can be beneficial in a variety of ways, from breathing techniques to pain management. I've yet to try unguided meditation since meditation is a new undertaking on my part that I began when I learned of the S.A.V.E.R.S.

ritual. The first S stands for Silence (aka meditation). When I practice the morning ritual, I try to allow 10–15 minutes for meditation, some days more, depending on the situation. If I'm in significant pain, especially from my eyes, I will spend more time on one of the pain management guided meditations I follow in the app "Breethe." There are many apps available for meditation for your Apple or Android devices. I have three different ones on my devices and switch back and forth depending on where I feel I could get the most benefit on any day. A few examples: as I write this paragraph this morning, I was pressed for time to do my ritual, so I condensed my usual hour for it in half—five minutes on each step. I woke up feeling little motivation to even get out of bed and especially write anything here, confronting every author's dread—writer's block.

The key to any meditation is breathing. Rhythmic breathing is what guided meditation coaches focus on most. It is a relaxation tool. The rhythm I find the best is the 4-4-6 method: inhale for a count of four, hold your breath for a count of four, then exhale for a count of six—a bit longer so you can expel all the air in your lungs before inhaling again. Repeat this several times, and it will help you relax. Relaxing your body helps open your mind to the suggestions and guidance of meditation itself. Your mind may wander, but that's okay. Acknowledge it and refocus during the breathing routine again for a few rounds. Take the time to explore the many mutual benefits of meditation—you'll be surprised.

- Read -

Read something that makes you happy. Avoid politics at all costs. Find a joke book, nature magazine, or something entirely out of the norm. I would even recommend, at the current state of the world, avoid reading the news at all costs because it can be detrimental to your health.

Pick up a book, anything you like or think you might like, even if it's a subject or genre you never considered before. Nothing or no one says you must read it cover to cover. If you don't like it, just put it down and pick another, or many others, until you find one that you like or that interests you. Feeding the mind is always a good thing, provided, of course, it benefits you. If what you are reading serves no good purpose, it's not worth wasting your time. If you are reading a book on how to build a bomb to make one and use it to cause harm, then that is for evil purposes and not good—don't do it!

Of course, reading is educational, you could learn something you maybe never knew before, or you may refine your knowledge or skills. It is also entertaining. One of my all-time favorite novels is *The Loneliness of the Long-Distance Runner* by Alan Sillitoe. The telling of the thoughts that went through the runner Smith's mind in the first-person was captivating for me as a teenager. While not an inmate in a reform school like Smith, I was, however, able to relate to him. My all-time favorite books were a series of mystery novels titled Alfred Hitchcock and the Three Investigators, about three teenage detectives. Once again, being a teenager myself, I could relate to some of the challenges they faced as adolescents, and I loved the mystery underlying their conquests. No matter your choice, reading stimulates the mind. If you read something that makes you laugh, you increase your mental, emotional, and physical benefits—that's even better! Getting lost in a book that captivates you is a wonderful way to escape the negatives in one's life.

- Daydream -

Daydream or discover something new. Stare out the window, clear your eyes, and go to the place of your dreams alone or with loved ones, where there is peace and joy in your very own private happy place. Look to see something you have never seen before, even if you have looked at the same scene a thousand times. As clouds drift by in the sky, imagine you are floating away on one, basking in the sense of freedom that would give you, floating in the boundless blue sky surrounding the earth.

Let your mind go places it's never been before—just let it wander and see where you go. When we were just kids, daydreaming was something only the lazy slackers did instead of their school assignments or chores. It was conveyed to us that daydreaming would never get us anywhere, and we wouldn't amount to much in life if we allowed it to become a regular practice. Oh, but to the contrary, daydreaming is now referred to as visualization or visualizing. It is now a recognized practice by the psychological community as a rewarding and motivating daily undertaking. Some of the most adept at this ritual are professional athletes. However, it is not limited to the pros alone, as they see themselves performing, rehearsing their game every step of the way, over and over in their minds, to perfect their performance for the upcoming competition.

It works. As an oarsman (also known as a rower) in high school, I would mentally rehearse each race the night before the regatta, visualizing every stroke of the oars from the starting line to the finish line. This ritual likely contributed to my early success, leading to my making the U.S. Junior National Team after just over a year in the sport. It was the first time I would wear a United States uniform. The next time would be as a U.S. Navy enlisted sailor and later as a commissioned officer—roles I also used to daydream (or visualize) about over and over until they became a reality.

For an even simpler version of daydreaming, let your mind drift away to a secluded island, a sandy beach, or a meadow with a babbling brook and fragrant flowers as far as the eye can see. Most importantly, ensure that your mental wanderings lead to a place of peace and happiness. Doing the opposite would be self-defeating and potentially emotionally disturbing. When I was younger, especially in my teenage years, with all the challenges that period can bring, my happy place was a hill overlooking the small town where I wished I had grown up instead of in the city of Philadelphia.

With my back against a mighty oak tree at the top of the hill, I would gaze down upon the quiet, peaceful town below, planning for my future, pondering the goings-on in the homes, offices, and stores before me, and wondering what the future held for me and the people below. A few years ago, I found the imaginary little town I used to watch from afar in my private daydreams. In reality, it is called Thurmont, Maryland. Driving through it for the first time on my way to a new job, I realized what this small town was, filling me with a wonderful sense of joy. Intriguingly, if I were to stand atop the mountain where I work, I could look down upon Thurmont. Regrettably, we have since moved to a different location. Find your happy place in your mind and take the time to visit it in your own daydreams as part of this ritual—enjoy and have a good time there!

- Set Goals -

Set a goal for yourself—becoming a professional actor, athlete, brain surgeon, dancer, millionaire, musician, President of the United States, professor, singer, or a Zamboni driver. Close your eyes and see yourself becoming just that, but most importantly, see the steps you must take to achieve your goal. The subconscious mind needs to adopt this quest to influence you with its powers; however, it must be conditioned through conscious thought before it can work its magic. First and foremost, once you have identified your desire, it must become a burning desire, and you must develop a plan for its attainment. Without said plan, achieving your goal will likely be elusive. Write your plan out and review it daily at night before going to sleep—when the subconscious mind is not clouded by the waking hour's influences of the conscious mind and is free to function at peak performance—and repeat that first thing in the morning. Make time here during this ritual to see yourself attaining that goal by rehearsing the steps of your plan as you visualize carrying them out.

Establish a mission for yourself, set a series of goals, write them down, use the S.M.A.R.T. (Specific, Measurable, Attainable, Relevant, and Time-bound) system, and read the plan aloud each day and night. Make it your mission in life. As Hal Elrod, author of the *Miracle Equation,* says, practice "unwavering faith" and "extraordinary effort," and you can achieve anything you set your mind to. Many of the great achievers have applied these very same principles and become mavens in their chosen pursuits.

- Discover Something New -

What awaits you if you take the time to disconnect from your devices and look around? Raise your chin, stop looking down at the world through a screen, and look up and around you. What do you see? There's an entire world out there, right in front of your eyes. Do you notice something you've never seen before? Can you look closer to understand what it is? Consider its color, size, shape, and whether it can move or make a sound. Is it animate or inanimate? Is it a living thing? What does it feel like? You can ask so many questions about something new, but first, you have to notice it—which is hard to do if a screen is constantly in your face. Your newfound discovery could change your life in the most positive ways.

For me, it was the first time I laid my eyes on a rowing shell. Although I had passed the Schuylkill River in Philadelphia at least a hundred times, I had not seen a rowing shell before. Then, on my second day of practice for my high school rowing team, I was introduced to every class of rowing shell in the Fairmount Rowing Association boathouse on famous Boathouse Row in Philadelphia. On the boat racks rested singles, doubles, pairs, quads, fours, and eights. All were made of wood, some Spanish cedar, and the grain from bow to stern was gorgeous and gleamed with a high gloss. I was captivated by their beauty.

Often, when rowing by myself in a single scull, the ripple of the water beneath the hull was musical, dulling the self-inflicted burn in every muscle of my body. Getting to row in them solidified my love affair with the sport, which led to my early success, competing in the Junior World Championships shortly after my first full year on the team. You don't have to take up a somewhat obscure elite sport such as crew, you have to take the time to look around you and not be buried in your device of choice.

- Listen to the World Beyond the Four Walls and Earbuds -

Step outside and listen to the sounds that fill the air. What do you hear? Today, we are bombarded 24-7-365 with noise. Not just noise from machines but the noise from the human talking heads—so-called experts—who tell you how to live your life and how you should think. You must listen to them if you are to be an accepted member of what their perception of humanity should be and how you must succumb to their will. Who do they think they are to tell me and you how to think and act? God Almighty? Nay, I say!

In my mind, one of the worst things to ever happen to society is the 24-hour news cycle, and it spawned the mass birth of these pundits to fill the 24 hours. The so-called "military experts" who always make me laugh and have never served a day in uniform in any military organization. Still, because they may have written a book on some military subject based solely on their research, they are now experts—phooey! Here's an even better one for you! Parenting experts who have never raised a child, but maybe just maybe, babysat a kid once, but they are going to tell me and you the best way to raise your child or children—again, I say phooey! Then you have the paid spokesperson who tells you the best thing to cure what ails you—phooey! Do you see a pattern here? We are bombarded day in and day out, 24/7, with tons of nonsense heaped on by so-called experts. At some point, you must grant yourself an escape—grab the remote fast—turn it off even for just five minutes a day and give yourself that reprieve. Go outside and listen to the sounds around you, whether it's the sounds of the city, a farm, a babbling brook, the ocean, or the sound of silence. Give your mind a breath of fresh air. It will do you wonders. Think happy thoughts, and you will reap the rewards many-fold!

- Raise Your Eyes to the Sky -

Look at what the Creator has put in place for you versus technology. I love the city skyline, especially at night, all aglow with thousands of lights. Then look out the window or up and down the street and take in the splendor of the scenery before your very own eyes. Someday, it could all be rubble, as were the beautiful cities of Europe after being bombed into destruction during World War II...don't miss out. Take the time to lift your head and look around you... you never know what you might discover!

Have you ever just stared up at the sky? There is something somewhat calming watching the clouds float up against that beautiful blue, but did you know there is also a psychological benefit to looking at that blue sky? There are many reasons. Research has been and still is being conducted worldwide by various people, from artists to students, into the benefits of staring at a blue sky, especially in the morning. As it turns out, there are multiple positive effects experienced, obvious and not so apparent, including psychological (obvious) from the sense of calm, serenity, and stability experienced, plus chemical (not so obvious) from the release of serotonin and cortisol within the body—even better if the sun is shining giving you a healthy dose of vitamin D. During the winter months, especially in some parts of the world where the days are repeatedly gray, a psychological effect called Seasonal Affective Disorder (SAD) causes depression for some people—a blue sky helps combat the effects of SAD.

The vastness of the sky alone promotes a sense of worth, hope, and realization of one's potential, as stated in the coined phrase, "the sky's the limit." From it stems inspiration that one can accomplish great things in their lifetime. The Wright brothers, Orville and Wilbur, used the sky to achieve greatness when they invented the flying machine that became the airplane. They looked up into the sky and saw the potential for a new form of transportation, utilizing the sky as its venue. Today, air travel is a multi-billion-dollar industry. Not only are people transported from one point on the globe to another thousands of miles apart, but so are goods and commodities via the wild blue sky. Orville and

Wilbur looked above and saw that man could fly—look into the vast blue and see what vision and inspiration may await you.

Watch as the clouds drift by in the sky and imagine you floating away on one with the sense of freedom that would give you in the boundless blue sky surrounding the earth.

Pull the plug now. You won't regret it!

STEP-4

GROW - Train Your Brain

*"[Humanity] has unquestionably one really effective weapon—
laughter…Against the assault of laughter nothing can stand."*
- Mark Twain

In Step-3 *Unplug*, the goal was to get you to put down the electronic device of choice and take in all around you that you miss with your head buried in the electronics daily.

One of the most potent human possessions at our disposal is the process of "autosuggestion." It is a way to train your mind, and it can have either positive or negative results. The most successful people in the world have trained their brains using this technique, as have some of the worst people humanity has ever known. In Napoleon Hill's book *How to Own Your Own Mind*, he learned from steel magnate Andrew Carnegie the enormous power of one's mind if trained properly through the application of several steps. These steps proved themselves repeatedly over time, as evidenced by the accomplishments of some of the most successful men on earth—Mr. Carnegie himself, Alexander Graham Bell, Thomas Edison, John Wannamaker, Henry T. Ford, and Woodrow Wilson, to name a few, each in their way.

Each of the men mentioned above combined the following tools to achieve their success: definiteness of purpose, the mastermind (explained later), applied faith, going the extra mile, organized individual endeavor, self-discipline, creative vision, organized thought, learning from defeat, inspiration, and attractive personality. The master-mind concept is one of the most significant. It requires the individual to assess their mental abilities. More importantly, it requires acknowledging areas where the person needs the assistance of people smarter than themselves. It takes a strong person to admit their shortcomings and an even stronger person to seek the help of others.

Through this brain training, a person's abilities to accomplish near-miraculous results are limited only by their self-imposed limitations. The 12 steps and the combination of five of them have led the men above to accomplish feats of which nations were saved (President Woodrow Wilson) and inventions created that opened ways to see in the dark (Thomas Edison) and converse across the globe (Alexander Graham Bell). I highly recommend reading Mr. Hill's book for the full explanations. It should be required in all high schools in the senior year.

Two of the processes require additional explanation, given they are closely linked and are the cornerstones of personal growth and success—"Definiteness of Purpose" and "Controlled Attention," according to Mr. Hill.

- Definiteness of Purpose: a motive, a burning desire obsessive in pursuing its attainment and the starting point of controlled (attention) habit; useless if not followed by intense action or effort.

Combined with:

- Controlled Attention: the major requirements being the will to succeed and a willingness to pay for the price of such achievement requiring no special abilities, education, or training, which can be achieved by any person with even average abilities.

Challenge your brain. What you can accomplish is solely up to you, if you put your mind to it. A sense of accomplishment is a wonderful realization and can bring a smile to your face and even a chuckle to your voice—and in turn, a feeling of happiness, not to mention all the benefits of laughing. Application of the two-step combination will provide you the way to unlimited personal success, regardless of your definition of success, provided they are used for good and not evil. However, you are wasting your time if you do not have a plan based on definiteness of purpose, written down, reviewed daily, and updated when necessary. Even worse, you may be wasting any talents you were imbued with.

- Learn Something New -

What is it you've always wanted to learn how to do but, for whatever reason, have yet to do so? Remember what it is? Please do it! Why not? What have you got to lose—a few bucks or a few hours? In the grand scheme of life, will it be worth a little sacrifice to learn that thing you have thought far too many times about but never took the time to pursue? Then do it! It could be life-changing! You may be amazed at what you can learn from all the knowledge for the taking. I've been reading books I always wanted to read, and the list is long and growing. Nonetheless, what I have read thus far is highly enlightening, and I am better off emotionally, financially, mentally, physically, and spiritually. Worth the time? *ABSOLUTELY!* Books alone are not the only source of education, although they are the cornerstone of learning and always will be.

YouTube is one of the best learning tools in our high-tech world these days, without question. Do you want to learn something new, how to fix something, how to clean between the two glass panes on your oven door? You name it, and you'll likely find it on YouTube. The terrific part is if you don't quite get it the first time you watch a how-to video, you can watch it as often as you need to. Even better, you can do so while you're trying to build, create, or fix whatever step-by-step using the pause button. No college lecture I attended ever had a repeat button on it, nor the visual aids like videos do—however, choose carefully.

- Do a Daily Puzzle -

Try a puzzle like Roku or the New York Times crossword. Hundreds of puzzle books are available on Amazon from $4.99 to over $20.00 each. There are hundreds of puzzles on the Internet, from crosswords to Wordscapes, and known as apps for your iPhone, iPad, or Android devices. Be kind to yourself if you are not an avid crossword or any mental puzzle aficionado. Start with something rated easy and work your way up to more difficult ones over time. If you start with a high degree of difficulty, you will likely end up frustrated or angry, and that is the exact opposite of what the goal of this step is—to enjoy what you are doing as you grow. Most importantly, don't cheat. That fails you more detrimentally than you realize, especially if you have any degree of conscience whatsoever. If you don't know the spelling of a particular word, pick up a dictionary and look it up—sorry, the old-timer in me came out—Google it.

- Do a Hand Puzzle -

Idle hands are the devil's workshop (or so the nuns told me in Catholic school). I am not sure about that, but working a physical hand puzzle increases dexterity and simultaneously challenges the mind. But, if it's frustrating, put it down for another time, or toss it in the trash if it's just plain pissing you off like the Rubik's Cube did to me—that's why it ceased to exist under a five-pound sledgehammer one night in the garage. I had to hit the damn thing five times, chasing it around the garage as it bounced away with each blow, trying to escape before it took its last breath in a hundred pieces, which of course, I had to sweep up. Hundreds of physical puzzles are available at various stores and on Amazon that will challenge you physically and mentally, so take the time to try one. If you don't like it, you can usually return it for a different one, or you can gift it to someone—the most aggravating ones to people you don't like!

- Take up a Hobby Requiring the Use of Your Hands -

To expand on the "idle hands" concept, there are literally thousands of things you can do with your hands that can prove worthwhile to yourself individually and mutually beneficial to others. Just as a few examples, auto mechanics is a skill where using the hands is essential. Even with the strides in robotics these days, there are just some places under the hood of a car where it takes a person's hands to access that nut or bolt. If you can repair your automobile, you have a skill that can aid others, especially in time of need. Woodworking is another skill requiring the use of one's hands. With such a skill, one could make toys to give to underprivileged children for Christmas—what a wonderful feeling that can be! Knitting requires using the hands to produce sweaters, scarves, and baby booties—a great talent. Not only are you training your brain, but you could also provide for others who may not be able to provide for themselves. In our world, those who help others reap benefits beyond monetary compensation gain a sense of self-worth. There's nothing wrong with that.

Training your brain can never be wasted time unless you do so for evil, as I previously stated. Learning to do something new is always positive and is another crucial ingredient in your overall happiness. Doing so each day in this five-step practice will be beneficial in more ways than one.

This leads me to the next and final of the five steps—Humor (me).

Ready to laugh some more? Read on!

HUMOR (me/us) - Make Someone Laugh

" The person who can bring the spirit of laughter
into a room is indeed blessed."
- Bennett Cerf

In Step 4, *Grow*, the goal was to get you to challenge your brain and learn something new, exercising those cells to better yourself mentally.

- Put a Smile on Someone's Face -

"Humor me," according to the "Amazing Talker[10]," means "a phrase that is used when someone wants someone else to do something, even though they may not want to do it or may not think it is necessary. It is often used to ask for a favor or a small indulgence, implying that the person asking is not taking the request too seriously and is just trying to be playful or lighthearted." It is also often used as a challenge to elicit additional information related to a particular claim or statement. Tell me more if what is being stated leaves a degree of doubt in the challenger's mind.

The word *humor* is defined in the Cambridge English Dictionary[11] as "to do what someone wants so that they do not become annoyed or upset." An example would be, "I ate the liver my wife cooked for dinner, even though I could have resoled my shoes with it, just to humor her."

I will use a different definition of "humor me." As I use it here in *Laugh Out Loud*, it means make me or anyone else laugh! C'mon, I triple-dog dare ya!

Making someone else laugh is as rewarding to yourself as it is to another.

Make someone else laugh by whatever means your heart desires:

- tell someone a joke

- play a harmless prank on someone—my favorite involves spooking someone, especially the wife, on Halloween. I'm partial to plastic/rubber spiders, snakes, and cockroaches around the house, in her pillow, in the freezer, or on the toilet seat

- wear something funny; post something humorous online (X (formerly Twitter), Facebook, Instagram, etc.)

- place/hang something funny where people will see it, use yourself as a prop to get a laugh

I love to make someone laugh. It makes me feel good that I can do so, especially given that I'm not that funny. To be totally transparent, I tell "dad jokes."

Having a sense of humor, I believe, is truly a gift God bestows on us. I've always felt it was sad that some people I've met lack that gift, not because it was denied but because they suppress it or don't realize they possess a sense of humor. Probably, in my feeble mind anyway, the best example of a human lacking, no, suppressing his sense of humor is Charles Dickens' Ebenezer Scrooge[12]. Downtrodden by life's pursuit of money and fortune, Scrooge became a bitter human who despised the young, old, rich, and poor. It took three ghosts, past, present, and future, for him to reflect on and examine his life, including the painful moments of it. The visitations prompted old Scrooge to come to his senses and change his life for the better, including exercising his sense of humor, stating in his own words, "I'm as merry as a schoolboy." What a wonderful feeling to be as merry as a schoolboy!

Have you ever had a laugh that stuck with you the rest of your life, something so funny it makes you laugh decades later? Take the time to remember that moment in your life from 10, 20, or 30 years ago, and let laughter take hold of you now. When you are done laughing, pause to recognize how good you feel right now—it's incredible, right?

In addition to my baby girl's belly laugh, I distinctly remember my son, Tim, blurted out a line at the dinner table that literally had me on the floor, tears streaming down my face from my laughter. He was looking at a photo I had come across when cleaning out my recently deceased father's house. It was me at about the age of four or five, standing with my grandmother, aunt, and uncle outside our house in Philly. It was some holiday, based on the manner of dress. Being the notorious streets of Philadelphia gunslinger I was at that age,

I had my hand cocked like a .357 Magnum pointing at the camera operator. This pose inspired my son, at 12, to mock me. As he looked at the photo, with his hand cocked like a pistol mimicking me, and in his best Edward G. Robinson gangster slang, he blurted out, "Take my picture again, and you'll be spitt'n bubblegum outta your forehead, see?" I lost it! His remark was perfect and delivered with the panache that any gangster back in the 1930s would relish—I think it was pickle relish I passed through my nose at that point. That was back in 1996. Every time I think of his declaration, I crack up even now, chronicling it here on this page. It feels good to relish in that memory—no pickles involved this time. It brings a smile to my face every time, a ray of sunshine into my heart, and a happy feeling in every cell in my body. All that from one 12-year-old wise guy remark. I'll take that all day, any day, especially on a bad day! I hope my son reads this memory and falls on the floor laughing, minus the pickle relish through the nose or bubblegum through his forehead.

Did that make you laugh? I hope so!

Did my experience trigger your memory of such a moment? Did it make you feel happy, even if for a fleeting moment? How good did that make you feel? Hold on to that moment for as long as you can! Let's take that feeling you just experienced and help someone else feel that way. I'm not kidding. It is mutually beneficial in more ways than you may think. Remember, in the chapter titled "It's a Process," I mentioned all the benefits of laughing. I'll repeat them here, so you don't have to go back to that chapter and end up losing your place here—one of my pet peeves—so here they are: beneficial reactions occur within the body that boosts numerous vital processes. Laughing is a:

- form of low-impact exercise that burns calories

- provides blood pressure regulation

- helps reduce pain

- provides increased oxygen (there's a good one), and

- gives a shot in the arm to the immune system.

How many doctors can do all that in one visit, plus there's no bill at the end of the month! Good luck if you decide to play doctor, make someone laugh, and then bill them for it! Hey, if you get away with it, let me know. I could use the extra cash!

If you lack a sense of humor or feel you do, develop one. It starts with a smile. Smile in the mirror; it may seem uncomfortable to smile at yourself, but do it anyway. Eventually, it will become much easier. Please try to smile at everyone you greet. It's reciprocal—one smile begets an equal reaction from the person you smile at, well, most of the time anyway. Please don't take the lack of a returned smile as a slight to you. The other person may have the worst day of their life. Your smile alone may be the one bright moment in another person's bad day. Practice smiling at yourself in the mirror, a trick *"Ma Bell[13]"* used to train telephone operators so they would sound pleasant. I'll bet that during this daily ritual, you'll laugh at yourself and think of the benefits in the previous paragraph!

Ready to discover what Laugh Out Loud can do for you, possibly even taking your life to the next level? Now, let's put it all together!

STARTING RIGHT NOW:
Laugh Out Loud - Live Happy & Enjoy Your Life

"Laugh often, long and loud. Laugh until you gasp for breath."
- George Carlin

I will revert to my education and training as an educator and instructor as I close out *Laugh Out Loud* and let you be on your way to experiencing the most fabulous dose of medicine ever known to humanity. As was hammered home to me in more than one classroom session, "Tell them what you're going to tell them—tell them—then tell them what you told them."

So, without further ado, this is the point where I tell you what I told you.

The sweetest sound in life is a child's laughter. There is nothing on this earth that can replace it. That sound alone can warm the heart of the most hardened of souls that have ever traversed the planet.

Laughter is more infectious than any pandemic ever grown in a lab as a weapon to eliminate human beings.

No bumbling idiot or his minions who occupy a position of utmost power can screw it up! No dictator can deny a single soul the right to chuckle, guffaw, giggle, or burst out in side-splitting laughter in their lifetime.

Laughter is resounding, so why not do it? Go ahead—*I triple-dog dare ya*—Laugh Out Loud!

It's also a choice, and the choice is entirely yours. Do you want to be happy, even just a little each day? Then, choose to be. It's up to you and you alone.

Here is where all five steps come together as a daily ritual, and remember, practice makes perfect. How you choose to implement and practice the following five (5) steps of the *Laugh Out Loud* ritual is also entirely up to you:

Step-1: *L*augh

Step-2: *A*ct

Step-3: *U*nplug

Step-4: *G*row

Step-5: *H*umor *(me/us)*

The five steps are designed to be completed in one hour, for an average of *12 minutes each (60 minutes divided by five steps)*. Any time, day or night!

Pressed for time, as we all are at what seems all too often these days, then you can knock out the five steps of *L*augh-*A*ct-*U*nplug-*G*row-*H*umor (me/us) (*L.A.U.G.H*) in five minutes, spending one minute on each. The benefits of even one minute per step will be beneficial if for no other reason than you step back from the toils of the day to take five minutes to come up for air, relax, and enjoy a good chuckle, guffaw, or giggle and de-stress. Take this mini vacation once daily or as many times as you need for your sanity and well-being.

The beauty of this daily ritual, and I highly recommend you make it a daily practice to reap its maximum benefits, is that it's flexible.

LAUGH - To Your Heart's Content

Having trouble thinking of something to make you laugh? Search Google, and you will find many funny things to get yourself chuckling. Another great place to look is in your TV listings; one of my favorite shows is "America's Funniest Videos"—it never disappoints. Then, there are various streaming services where you can find a comedy movie or stand-up routines.

Whatever you choose, allow yourself to laugh until you cry—it's healthy for you!

CAUTION/DISCLAIMER: Do not do Step-1 Laugh—while eating, you could be a new statistic, the evening news headline reading, they died laughing (and choked to death) eating a ham sandwich (with mustard and pickles)—and I go to jail for killing you with laughter! That's unhealthy for both of us!

ACT - Get Your Blood Flowing

CAUTION/DISCLAIMER: As with any exercise, you must be aware of your limitations, especially if you have any underlying health conditions that would make exercising potentially harmful to your overall well-being. If in doubt, consult your physician for guidance. Even the laughing exercises described below could need your doctor's advice. Also, depending upon where you are, you may have to consider your safety if venturing beyond your home's or other dwelling's security.

The goal is to move your body and exercise your muscles and lungs. However, you choose to do so is entirely your choice. If you currently live a sedentary lifestyle or are stuck behind a desk all day, the benefits of regular recurring exercise are invaluable. Exercise does not need to be strenuous for you to reap the rewards. If you don't currently exercise regularly, starting slowly and building up to a goal you have set for yourself is highly advised. The first several days will be challenging, but if you follow this practice, it will get easier, and you'll be able to laugh off the pain.

UNPLUG - Put the Darn Device Down

Turn off the devices, iPhones, iPads, iWatches, Androids, cell phones, TVs, radios, and so on.

Daydream or discover something new. Stare out the window, clear your eyes, and go to the place of your dreams alone or with loved ones, where there is peacefulness and joy in your private happy place. Watch as the clouds drift by in the sky and imagine you are floating away on one with the sense of freedom that would give you in the boundless blue sky that surrounds the earth.

Meditation is a great way to escape from the world around you and allow your mind to relax from all the stress it is required to endure in today's world.

How about a stroll through a park or sitting on the beach, listening to the beautiful sounds around you and not some talking head spewing bad news, nonsense, or hatred?

GROW - Train Your Brain

You're never too old to learn, so why not challenge your brain each day—what's there to lose? With the built-in flexibility of this daily ritual, you can dedicate 60 seconds or several minutes (12) to learning something new. Take time to improve your knowledge of whatever you desire—the opportunities are limitless. There are no limits beyond those you self-impose.

Learning a new skill may be life-changing for you—the stories are many from around the globe. Discovering a hidden talent could very well turn out to be your golden ticket to fame and fortune. Please remember me if you do hit it rich.

What you can accomplish is solely up to you. A sense of accomplishment is a wonderful realization that can bring a smile and even a chuckle to your voice.

HUMOR (me/us) - Make someone laugh

I will use a different definition of "humor me"—as I use it here in *Laugh Out Loud*, it means make me or anyone else laugh! C'mon, I triple-dog dare ya!

Making someone else laugh is as rewarding to yourself as it is to another. When you can laugh at yourself, you have achieved a state of happiness. When you make others laugh, you have shared a gift more valuable than any gold coin or gemstone.

My final anecdote. When my youngest daughter Erin was still a baby—about 12–15 months old—I would wheel her around in her stroller in the Navy Commissary or Exchange at Naval Air Station Miramar, California, north of San Diego. As her mother browsed the variety of goods and goodies, I engaged my little wee one in serious debates, yes, debates. To keep her occupied and not fussing, I would ask her questions like, "So, Miss Erin, what do you think about the current state of the U.S. economy?" To which she replied, with absolute gibberish and cooing, but with utmost conviction and her honest, highly educated, worldly experienced opinion. Once I got her started, she was on a roll. "But Erin, how could you make such a statement given the current Gross Domestic Product numbers?" Once again, her highly experienced retort with even more conviction rolled off her lips with acumen.

Anyone within earshot was laughing at the ongoing debate and typically commented, "She's quite the astute little businesswoman and so cute, too." I'm sure a few of those who listened went home and conveyed the story of the debate between the father and his baby titan of Wall Street. Mission accomplished: we made someone laugh!

Remember that laughter is contagious. It's the best medicine on earth, bar none! The benefits of laughter are numerous to body, mind, and soul. Having a good laugh, especially with another, helps put smiles on your faces, a ray of sunshine in your hearts, and a moment of happiness in your lives—what could possibly be wrong with that?

- Time to Get Started -

Take the time to test the five steps for yourself.

Well, whadda, ya think? Not bad, huh? Did you laugh even for a few seconds? How'd it make you feel? Good right?! Now go ahead and repeat Step-1. *Laugh again just because you can!*

Happiness is a choice. Whether or not you choose to be happy is entirely up to you. No one else can make that decision for you. Things can occur in your life and even pile up beyond your comprehension. Regardless, practice this ritual, and you will be able to smile and laugh again, which will help you deal with life one chuckle at a time—trust me, I know. The potential transformation of practicing the five steps can be eye-opening and life-changing. Just being able to laugh proved lifesaving for me.

If you have arrived at this point in *Laugh Out Loud*, I want to thank you with my sincerest gratitude for putting your faith in me to read this little ditty I've written. It has been a labor of love and hopefully will become a symbol of my love for humanity and belief that there are good people on this earth. We don't hear enough about them day to day.

Don't forget to pre-register at the beginning of the book for your free audiobook version of *Laugh Out Loud* and your discounted copy of *Blind Treason*.

THIS IS IT
LAUGH OUT LOUD!

"BLIND TREASON"
INTRODUCTION

I had just told the Defense Security Service agent, the one I told the day before over the phone had to contact my lawyer and commanding officer before I would talk to him, to take a hike and threatened to have him escorted out, wondering how he made it to the 10th floor and my desk without an escort. I cracked a joke as he waddled away. Kevin, who sat six feet from my desk, asked, "Jack, how do you do it, man?"

"Do what?" I retorted.

"Keep a sense of humor with all the bullshit you've had to deal with since getting shot with the laser?" he inquired.

"I find something to laugh at. If I don't laugh, I will cry, and my eyes will only hurt worse than they always do," I responded.

Yes, you read the previous question from Kevin correctly. I was shot in the face with a laser from a Russian spy ship on April 4th, 1997, near Seattle, Washington. I was flying in a Canadian Air Force CH-124 Sea King helicopter, taking photographs of a Russian cargo vessel that U.S. Naval Intelligence, for which I worked, suspected of working on behalf of Russian military intelligence, the GRU, and the

Federal Security Bureau (FSB) (formerly the KGB). My eyes were burned by the laser fired at us that day, and my retinas still bear the scars today. However, as the game is played in the intelligence business, what I just told you... never happened. The often-mind-numbing pain I have lived with every day for the last 26 plus years is only in my imagination, per the United States Navy and Department of Defense. To prove them wrong, the full tell-all story will be revealed in my upcoming book, *"BLIND TREASON, The True-Life Story of Survival of an American Spy Left Out in the Cold."*

A half-off coupon and a website link to pre-order a copy can be found at the end of this introduction.

There are more Russian spies operating in the United States today than during the height of the Cold War, and Vladimir Putin is doing everything in his power to turn the U.S. into a Communist State. He's experiencing success. It is only a matter of time unless we wake up and stop what is happening. In 1989, the destruction of the Berlin Wall supposedly signified the final nail in the coffin of Communism in the Soviet Union, and the world breathed a sigh of relief as politicians and pundits alike proclaimed that the Cold War had finally come to an end. However, the shadowed reality of our world and the true relationship shared between the United States and the Russian Federation lie in stark contrast to the peaceful, cooperative image postulated by the global media and our nation's leaders.

The facts are alarming. A former KGB spy leads Russia, our major cities remain targeted by Russian nuclear missiles, and Vladimir Putin threatens to use them. Inexpensive Russian weapons are in mass circulation on the Black Market, and covert Cold War spy games are still taking place on a massive level. These facts have been watered down and obscured for the American public in the name of economic cooperation and political gain. In some cases, the government's efforts to hide the truth have evolved into full-blown conspiracies and blatant cover-ups. But would the United States government go so far as to cover up an act of war in United States territory? Would our trusted politicians and military elite attempt to silence, discredit, and destroy the unblemished record of a highly praised American Naval Intelligence Officer wounded in the line of duty? The disturbing reality is yes, they would, and yes, they have.

This shocking exposé is based on the author's 15 years of experience in defense intelligence and his own first-hand experience battling the intelligence apparatus of the former Soviet Union et al. *Blind Treason* will be the complete story of Russia's unprovoked, April 4th, 1997, attack on the United States and Canada, and how the author, a veteran United States Navy Intelligence Officer, and a Canadian Air Force helicopter pilot were both permanently wounded, abandoned, and betrayed for underhanded political reasons. It will also tell the story of how being wounded during the attack with a sophisticated, secret laser weapon would eventually save one of their lives and forever change the way military pilots carry out their missions. Further evidence will show that lasers are also being used against commercial airline pilots and can easily be used by terrorists at any time and place, with no way to identify those responsible.

Blind Treason will reveal now-declassified government secrets of how the United States and Canada came under a Russian attack in United States' airspace just five nautical miles from American shores. It will also expose the Government cover-up that continues to this day, denying the attack ever took place. This is a true story of survival through a painful "David and Goliath" battle that pitted a career United States Navy spy against the President of the United States and his treasonous lieutenants. At stake—the National Security of our country.

Blind Treason will reveal the corrupt efforts undertaken at the White House, State Department, Pentagon, and government facilities across North America to deny that this act of war ever occurred and to discredit the man who swore an oath to the *People* of the United States, to "protect and defend (them) against all enemies foreign and domestic." Any American who reads *Blind Treason* will be appalled at how a President, his Administration, and the United States Navy sacrificed one of its own to avoid tarnishing our "friendly" relationship with Russia, an enemy still to this day.

It has long been the necessary duty of the United States to gather and maintain intelligence on all threats that arise in the world to protect its people and the citizens of foreign nations. In this age of global terrorism, our intelligence efforts are more critical than ever. Yet, over two decades ago, an American Intelligence Officer was the victim of an act of war while performing his duty, and our government turned its back on him. This betrayal shall not go unnoticed. Every American deserves to know the truth so that history can accurately reflect upon those who stood to uphold liberty and justice and those who sought to exploit it. In *Blind Treason*, the truth shall be revealed. *Blind Treason* will be the first book to prove that the Cold War never ended.

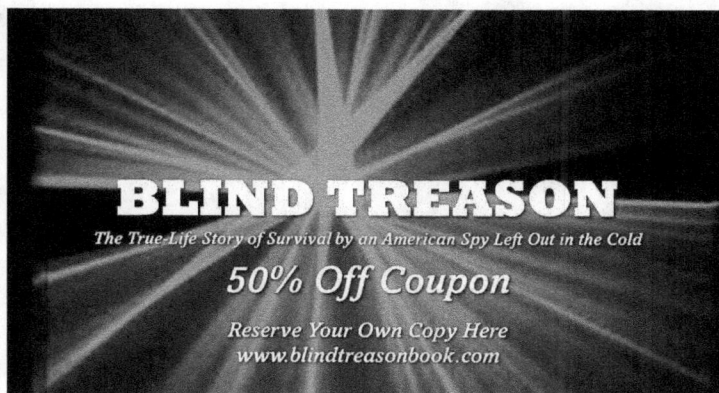

BLIND TREASON

The True-Life Story of Survival by an American Spy Left Out in the Cold

50% Off Coupon

Reserve Your Own Copy Here
www.blindtreasonbook.com

DISCLAIMER: The views expressed in this publication are those of the author and do not necessarily reflect the official policy or position of the Department of Defense or the U.S. government. The public release clearance of this publication by the Department of Defense does not imply Department of Defense endorsement or factual accuracy of the material.

Resources

505 Best of Laughter Exercises (https://tinyurl.com/505-Best-Laughter-Exercises)

Alfred Hitchcock and the Three Investigators (https://tinyurl.com/Laugh-Out-Loud-3-Investigators)

Boathouse Row (https://en.wikipedia.org/wiki/Boathouse_Row)

Foster Brooks (https://tinyurl.com/Laugh-Out-Loud-Foster-Brooks)

Jokes of the Day (https://tinyurl.com/Laugh-Out-Loud-Jokes-of-Day)

Jonathan Winters (https://tinyurl.com/Laugh-Out-Loud-JWinters)

Laughter Online University (LOU) (https://www.laughteronlineuniversity.com/)

Robin Williams (https://tinyurl.com/Laugh-Out-Loud-Robin-Williams)

Rose in her car seat (https://tinyurl.com/Laugh-Out-Loud-Rose-Car-Seat)

Seven Words You Can Never Say on Television (https://tinyurl.com/Laugh-Out-Loud-Seven-Words)

The Confessional   (https://tinyurl.com/
Laugh-Out-Loud-Confessional)

The Far Side (https://www.thefarside.com)

The Miracle Morning (https://miraclemorning.com/books/)

Tim Conway (https://tinyurl.com/
Laugh-Out-Loud-Tim-Conway)

Toys for Tots (https://www.toysfortots.org/)

Who's on First? (https://tinyurl.com/
Laugh-Out-Loud-Whos-On-First)

Acknowledgments

I want to pass to the below listed folks my sincerest heartfelt THANK YOU for aiding me on this journey!

Andrea Daly – my behind-the-scenes support structure and biggest cheerleader!

Hal Elrod – thank you for providing me the inspiration.

Chandler Bolt, Sean Sumner, and Scott Allen – my coaching staff who showed me how.

The Self-Publishing Team – from account establishment to finished product – what a team!

Sebastian Gendry – for your supportive words.

Justin Cremisio – thanks for your encouragement boss!

Last but by no means least – My Launch Team – you are the ones who got me over the finish line!

Author Bio

JACK DALY

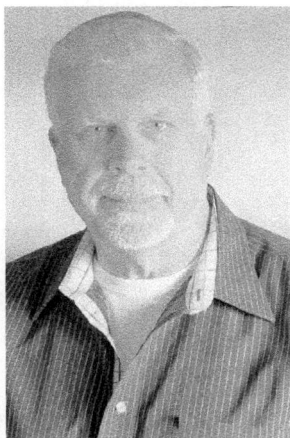

Jack Daly is a native of Philadelphia, Pennsylvania, and a retired U.S. Naval Officer with over 20 years of service to his country in various assignments, including aviation, surface and amphibious warfare, communications, and intelligence. Jack's first time wearing a United States uniform, Red, White, and Blue, came at the end of his senior year in high school in 1976 when he represented the United States at the Junior World Rowing Championships in the double-scull (2x) event. During his enlisted days, Jack completed his bachelor's degree and received his commission via Officer Candidate School in Newport, Rhode Island. Jack works as an Emergency Management Specialist within the Department of Defense today.

Repeated disturbing reports of daily military and veteran suicides prompted Jack to try to find a way to help all those struggling or troubled emotionally. Add the COVID-19 pandemic and strife worldwide, the need proved even more significant. Based on his experience, Jack found a proven tool that worked every time he needed it—laughter—thus the writing of *Laugh Out Loud*.

Thank You for Reading My Book!

I really appreciate all your feedback and I love hearing what you have to say.

Please take two minutes now to leave a helpful review on Amazon, let me know what you thought of the book:

www.laughoutloudbook.com/review

Thanks so much!
Jack Daly

References

1   Wilson, Kim, Kelly Candaele, and Lowell Ganz. 1992. A League of Their Own. Comedy, Drama, Sport. Directed by Penny Marshall. United States: N/A. N/A.

2   Berk, Lee S., Stanley A. Tan, William F. Fry, Barbara J. Napier, Jerry W. Lee, Richard W. Hubbard, John E. Lewis, and William C. Eby. 1989. "Neuroendocrine and Stress Hormone Changes During Mirthful Laughter - ScienceDirect." ScienceDirect.Com | Science, Health and Medical Journals, Full Text Articles and Books. The American Journal of the Medical Sciences, Volume 298, Issue 6. 1989, https://www.sciencedirect.com/science/article/pii/S0002962915361929, Pages 390-396, ISSN 0002-9629.

3   "Stress Relief from Laughter? It's No Joke - Mayo Clinic." 2023. Mayo Clinic. September 22, 2023. https://www.mayoclinic.org/healthy-lifestyle/stress-management/in-depth/stress-relief/art-20044456.

4   Underlined names and terminology in the paperback version have URL links in the Resources section at the back of the book.

5   "Books by Hal Elrod – Multiple Amazon Best Sellers." n.d. The Miracle Morning. Accessed November 21, 2023. https://miraclemorning.com/books/.

6   Gendry, Sebastian. 2012. "Funny Fitness Is Really Good For You!" Laughter Online University. https://www.facebook.com/sebastiangendry/. January 10, 2012 https://www.laughteronlineuniversity.com/laughter-fitness/.

7   "505 Best of Laughter Exercises." n.d. Laughter Online University. Accessed November 21, 2023. https://www.laughteronlineuniversity.com/store/books/best-of-laughter-exercises/.

8   Administration, National Highway Traffic Safety. 2023. "Traffic Safety Facts Distracted Driving in 2021, DOT HS 813 443." Department of Transportation/NHTSA. U.S. Department of Transportation. 2023. https://crashstats.nhtsa.dot.gov/#!/PublicationList/41.

9   Hill, Napoleon. 2018. How to Own Your Own Mind. Prabhat Prakashan.

10   "What Does 'Humor Me' Mean? How to Use It?" 2022. AmazingTalker. December 19, 2022. https://tw.amazingtalker.com/questions/1307.

11   Cambridge Dicitionary. © Cambridge University Press & Assessment 2023, https://dictionary.cambridge.org/us/dictionary/english/humor, humor definition

12   Dickens, Charles. 1843. A Christmas Carol. First. London: Chapman & Hall.

13   "Bell System History - The Bell System." n.d. Bell System Memorial Home Page. Accessed November 21, 2023. https://www.bellsystemmemorial.com/bellsystem_history.html.

selfpublishing.com

NOW IT'S YOUR TURN

Discover the EXACT 3-step blueprint you need to become a bestselling author in as little as 3 months.

Self-Publishing School helped me,
and now I want them to help you
with this FREE resource to begin outlining your book!
Even if you're busy, bad at writing, or don't know where to
start,you CAN write a bestseller and build your best life.
With tools and experience across a variety of niches and
professions,Self-Publishing School is the only resource you
need totake your book to the finish line!

DON'T WAIT
Say "YES" to becoming a bestseller:
https://selfpublishing.com/friend/

Follow the steps on the page to get a FREE resource to get
started on your book and unlock a discount to get started
with SelfPublishing.com